Frequently

all about
ginseng

STEPHEN FULDER, PhD

AVERY PUBLISHING GROUP
Garden City Park • New York

The information contained in this book is based upon the research and personal and professional experiences of the author. They are not intended as a substitute for consulting with your physician or other health care provider. Any attempt to diagnose and treat an illness should be done under the direction of a health care professional.

The publisher does not advocate the use of any particular health care protocol, but believes the information in this book should be available to the public. The publisher and author are not responsible for any adverse effects or consequences resulting from the use of any of the suggestions, preparations, or procedures discussed in this book. Should the reader have any questions concerning the appropriateness of any procedure or preparation mentioned, the author and the publisher strongly suggest consulting a professional health care advisor.

Series cover designer: Eric Macaluso
Cover image courtesy of The Steven Foster Group

ISBN: 0-89529-892-9

Printed in the United States of America

10   9   8   7   6   5   4   3

Contents

Introduction, 5

1. Panacea or Pick-Me-Up?, 9
2. Ginseng, Energy, and Vitality, 19
3. How to Boost Performance, 31
4. Ginseng and Stress, 41
5. Young Body, Young Mind, 57
6. Ginseng's Myth, Legend, and History, 67
7. Buying and Using Ginseng, 75

Conclusion, 83

Glossary, 85
References, 87
Suggested Readings, 89
Index, 91

Introduction

Do you feel tired? Stressed-out? Are you often overwhelmed by the many demands upon your time and your energy? If your answer to these questions are yes, then you are not alone. Most Americans go through periods of exhaustion, tension, and even burn-out, as they attempt to juggle numerous complicated commitments, including family, work, and recreation. The stressful struggle to balance the components of life in an increasingly complex world often contributes to health problems. Indeed, it would be fair to say that stress has reached epidemic proportions in the Western world and is responsible for some debilitating illnesses, as well as many chronic, nagging health problems.

It is exactly for such health problems that we must turn to natural herbal remedies. These products are excellent for those daily life situations in which we find ourselves not sick, but not healthy either. And where tiredness and stress are concerned, there is one remedy that stands out: ginseng. Ginseng is so effective that I am fond of calling it "the root of power."

Ginseng is probably the best known of all Oriental herbs. Millions of people all over the world take it daily to boost their energy, vitality, and performance or in special situations such as convalescence, aging, and recovery. It has become the main tonic herb in the West, just as it was in the East for thousands of years. It is available in most pharmacies and has now been included in many of the official drug guides of European countries.

In *All About Ginseng*, you will meet this root, known scientifically as *Panax ginseng*. Your imagination and sense of mystery will be tickled, because the ginseng root is shaped like a human being. Perhaps because of its interesting and human shape, there is a great deal of legend, folklore, and superstition associated with ginseng—as well as a great deal of misunderstanding. But there is nothing fanciful or superstitious about the effectiveness of this extraordinary herb. Scientific research— some of which I have personally conducted—provides ample support to the claim that ginseng is a powerful and useful herb to combat stress and fatigue, to maximize stamina, and to build strength.

This book will answer your most basic questions about ginseng. You will discover what it really is, what it contains, and where it comes from. We will address and dispel misunderstandings and myths surrounding ginseng, and explain what it can and cannot do to improve your health and vitality. You will learn how to use ginseng to combat fatigue and improve performance, and why ginseng is a more healthful and effective substance than other stimulants or body-builders that you might have taken in the past. You'll learn how to use ginseng in demanding situations such as sports, examinations, jet lag, insufficient sleep, and when you are feeling low. You'll find out if ginseng really is an aphrodisiac, as many people have claimed.

By the time you have finished reading this book, you will realize that you have a powerful and potent ally to help you through life's stresses so that instead of feeling exhausted and overwhelmed, you feel alert, energetic, strong, and capable of meeting your many commitments successfully and in good health.

1.

Panacea or Pick-Me-Up?

Ginseng is a root of a plant that is described in the poetic language of the Orient as the ultimate panacea. Years ago, it was enormously expensive, very exotic, and hard to obtain. Today, it is far more easily accessible and is used all over the world as a tonic remedy. In this chapter, you will learn what ginseng is, what it can do for you, and where it comes from. You will also learn something about the history of this fascinating herb—its background in Oriental medicine and how it arrived in the West.

Q. What can ginseng do for me?

A. Ginseng is a unique herb that is regarded in Eastern medicine as the most precious of all traditional remedies. Its popularity is no longer confined to the Orient. Indeed, it has become quite popular in the West as well. It can give you extra energy and vitality, particularly in many situations of stress and exhaustion.

Ginseng has both short-term and long-term uses. On a short-term basis, you can use ginseng as a rapid and safe stimulant if you've had a sleepless night, if you must cope with an unusually heavy work load, if you're a student facing final exams, if you're suffering from jet lag, or if you wish to improve your performance during an important sports game. Ginseng can also be used to address long-term problems—for example, in recovering from periods of stress and burn-out, in convalescence, in intensive sports training, and in generally remaining alert if you know you are going through an extended period of high stress accompanied by many physical or emotional demands. Ginseng can improve your sexual performance. It is not an aphrodisiac, in the sense of being a sexual stimulant; however it can help to maintain sexual energy and may also help in cases of impotence.

Q. Why take ginseng when I'm tired if I can drink coffee?

A. Ginseng isn't just a stimulant. It is a tonic—in fact, it is probably the only true tonic available today. Ginseng works differently from caffeine. It does not produce instant wakefulness which is paid for by even more exhaustion later. Its real value is that it increases vitality and performance, while at the same time improving your health. Caffeine, on the other hand, cannot truly increase vitality and help you overcome stress, exhaustion, or burn-out. It is a "quick-fix" remedy that comes with a very heavy price tag once its immediate effects have worn off.

Ginseng does more than simply helping you cope with tiredness, as caffeine does. It can also help your body cope with almost every other kind of stress. A large number of scientific studies have confirmed that ginseng can prevent the harmful effects of stress on your body. If you are under continuous stress, or you drive yourself too hard and don't make time for relaxation, the continuous state of inner tension can increase blood pressure and cholesterol, and damage your immunity and your health. Ginseng can help you to prevent these changes. It can protect your immunity and shield your general inner balance from stress-related damage. It is also an excellent anti-aging remedy that can be taken regularly to help prevent the decline in energy and vitality that so often accompanies the aging process.

Q. Can ginseng actually cure any diseases?

A. Ginseng is not a drug like penicillin, for example, that treats a specific disease. It addresses certain symptoms, such as fatigue and weakness, but it is more helpful in building health and vitality, and in helping the body cope with stress and tiredness, both of which take a serious toll on the immune system.

Q. So what exactly is ginseng?

A. Ginseng is the root of a small herb. Its botanical, or scientific name is *Panax ginseng*. Botanists gave it the name "Panax," which is Latin for "panacea," because the Oriental peoples regard it as a panacea, or a cure-all. "Ginseng" comes from the Chinese word for "root of man".

Ginseng belongs to the small family called the *Araliaceae*, which includes sarsaparilla and ivy. For such a famous plant, it looks remarkably humble. It has groups of five saw-toothed leaves atop a long, straight stalk, which may be about eight to thirty inches tall, depending on age. Its pale green flowers begin to appear only when the plant is two or three years old. These produce bright red berries, well-liked by people and birds. Ginseng grows in the shade in cold climates, and the above-ground parts die off every winter. New growth starts from buds on the "neck" of the root every spring.

The medicinal part of ginseng is the thick, fleshy root. It is somewhat like a carrot but yellow, not orange. It has many tendrils and rootlets, and may sometimes be branched, curled, or bent. The fresh root tastes somewhat bitter, with a hint of aromatic sweetness.

Asian ginseng once grew naturally in the shaded high temperate forests of China, Korea, Japan, and the Eastern part of the former USSR, but it is now virtually extinct in its wild state. However, cultivation has spread the domesticated ginseng to many other areas in Eastern Asia. Although the Chinese undoubtedly value the wild ginseng above any other plant, they regard even the cultivated variety as their most important medicine.

Q. Are there other important types of ginseng besides the Asian ginseng?

A. Yes. The closest cousin to Asian ginseng is American ginseng, which grows wild and is cultivated in the northern United States, particularly Wisconsin, and in Canada. It is described botanically as *Panax quinquefolium*. It looks like a compact version of Asian ginseng and was famous as a medicine among the North American Indians. American ginseng is not much used in Western countries, but is exported to China where it is appreciated as an alternative to Asian ginseng. It is somewhat different from Asian ginseng, as we'll see below. Asian ginseng is the only ginseng available in the United States today.

There are also some other species, including Himalayan ginseng, and San ch'i ginseng, which are similar to Asian ginseng and are used in traditional medicine. However, they are not available in the West.

Q. What is Siberian ginseng?

A. Siberian ginseng isn't actually ginseng at all. Its scientific name is *Eleutherococcus*, or *eleuthero* for short. It has mistakenly been called "ginseng" because it has similar effects to actual ginseng: it is a powerful tonic and energy-provider. So-called "Siberian ginseng" is a spiny bush that grows in Eastern Russia and China. It was introduced by the Russians as an alternative to true ginseng, because the true ginseng had become expensive and difficult to supply. It is well-known as a tonic in traditional medicine of Russia and China.

Q. What makes ginseng work so well?

A. Ginseng contains a unique range of chemical substances called ginsenosides. They have a chemical structure that resembles the hormones (chemical messengers) that the human body uses to organize the reactions to stress. Studies have shown that ginsenosides increase the stamina, recovery, and resistance to stress in animals who have engaged in long periods of forced exercise.

Ginseng contains other important constituents as well. For example, certain starchy substances in the root appear to help the immune system, while others are involved assisting the body to break down sugar and convert it into energy.

Q. Why was ginseng described as a panacea?

A. The word panacea means "all-healing". It has come to mean a medicine that can cure any illness. This term was incorrectly applied to ginseng by the first Westerners who visited China. They heard the wildly extravagant praises bestowed on the ginseng root by the Chinese and assumed that ginseng could cure anything. But the Chinese never claimed that ginseng is a panacea, only that it has extraordinary abilities to enhance health, vitality, and energy. This is one of many misunderstandings about ginseng that the Western world has held for many years.

Q. Are the effects of ginseng psychological or physical?

A. The powerful effects of ginseng are physical. At one time, the conventional medical world regarded ginseng (and most other herbs) with skepticism and even downright derision. An early edition of the *United States National Formulary* (the official governmental drug guide) said that the "medical properties of ginseng . . . had no other existence than in the minds of the Chinese." An early edition of the *Encyclopedia Britannica* called ginseng "a worthless plant."

Ginseng was misunderstood by doctors and scientists because it did not conform to the conventional understanding of drugs. Researchers are accustomed to the modern view that regards a drug as a single substance designed to treat a single symptom, like a headache, or acts on a single biological process, such as blood pressure. A remedy used by essentially healthy people to increase energy and enhance health is unfamiliar to modern medicine, and its effects are hard to measure in the laboratory. However from the perspective of Chinese medicine, a remedy that does not cure a disease, but brings health and vitality, is very precious indeed, because it can help to prevent ill health. This Oriental perspective has not always been understood in the West.

In recent years, the Western medical view of ginseng has begun to change. Today, a major multinational pharmaceutical company is involved in producing ginseng products. Ginseng is listed in many of the official drug guides of Europe and other countries and is available in most pharmacies. There are more than 2,000 scientific studies demonstrating that ginseng has genuine tonic and stress-preventing effects. These studies have gone a long way in convincing responsible modern doctors that ginseng really does work, especially since some of these studies have been performed on animals. It is fair to assume that laboratory animals whose health improves as a result of ginseng are not experiencing improvement because of psychological reasons!

2.

Ginseng, Energy, and Vitality

The most important use of ginseng is as an energy-booster. In this chapter we will discuss what ginseng can do for your energy levels. You will learn about an array of circumstances in which ginseng can be useful, how to take it to cope with tiredness and exhaustion, whether it will increase energy even if you're not tired, and why it is superior to other common stimulants such as caffeine.

Q. What is the main use of ginseng?

A. Ginseng increases energy and vitality when you feel that you need a boost. It is ideal for those situations when you feel depleted, wake up tired, have low motivation or mild depression, and lack "get up and go." Ginseng will be helpful whatever the reason for your low energy level—whether it is just generalized tension, excessive amounts of food or sex, too little or too much exercise, lack of sleep, overwork, or emotional conflicts with people around you.

Q. Doesn't that make ginseng a stimulant, like caffeine?

A. Ginseng certainly is a stimulant, but it is quite different from coffee, as mentioned in the last chapter. If you drink a cup of coffee, you feel its effects immediately. When the effects of the caffeine have worn off, you're even more tired than you were before, and you hasten to drink another cup so that you can function effectively. Many people experience a distressing "crash" when the effects of coffee have worn off.

Ginseng works differently. If you take ginseng when you are tired, you will not feel the immediate surge of energy that you would get from a cup of coffee, nor do you experience a crash several hours later. The effects of ginseng build up over time, and the sense of vigor and strength increase. Regular use of ginseng will lead you to a healthy level of energy that you can sustain. For this reason, ginseng is not described as a stimulant but rather as a tonic—a substance that invigorates and strengthens.

Q. Have scientists investigated the differences between coffee and ginseng?

A. Scientific research has explored the differences between stimulants and ginseng and found out that stimulants hasten the breakdown of energy that is stored in the body. This leads to a quick peak of sugar in the blood. In contrast, ginseng seems to improve how the body burns sugar. There are studies by Professor Oura and others at the University of Tokyo, showing that ginseng helps the cells to take in sugar from the blood and use it more effectively. I myself have conducted studies together with Dr. Deepak Shori at London University. We demonstrated that if animals were given ginseng, their brain cells utilized necessary nutrients more efficiently.

A cup of coffee now and then can be helpful as a short-term stimulant, and most of use and enjoy it as part of our daily life. But if we rely on caffeine to give us energy, we find that in the long run it does the reverse. It actually decreases our energy. Caffeine creates a rapid surge of energy and alertness. It works by generating additional release of adrenalin in the body. The adrenalin raises blood sugar levels and thereby increases the body's available fuel, creating an energy surge. Unfortunately, that process carries a serious price tag. It is enormously stressful to the body. It reduces overall health and adds to exhaustion in the long term. It is like living on an overdraft from the bank; the interest accumulates, and in the end the credit runs out. The body's energy reserves are used up and not replaced.

Ginseng functions in an different way. It is not a stimulant which generates short-term alertness at the expense of long-term health. Quite the opposite. Ginseng increases health instead of decreasing it. Unlike coffee and other stimulants, which attack your health over time, ginseng builds your health over time. The longer you use it, the better you feel. Ginseng fills the pool of energy so that there is more available, while stimulants drain it.

Perhaps most important of all, ginseng is not addictive. If you miss a day or two of ginseng, you are unlikely to experience the exhaustion, irritability, and headaches that often accompany caffeine withdrawal.

Q. Will ginseng correct all my health problems, since I don't have time to really take care of myself?

A. No, ginseng in not a "magic bullet," and it

won't compensate for total abuse or neglect of your health. However, ginseng can reduce the damage that an unhealthy lifestyle inflicts upon your body. For example, if your diet is poor, and you eat a great deal of processed food, fats, and empty calories, or if you do not take any exercise, you may feel tired. In this case, tiredness is a symptom of poor health. Ginseng will help to reduce the tiredness, and it will even help the body to cope with the stress of poor living, to a certain extent. But it will not solve the basic problem, and the symptoms of tiredness will eventually return. So you should view ginseng as an aid to help you cope, while simultaneously dealing with health problems by introducing other appropriate self-care measures into your life.

Q. Can it help with insomnia and jet lag?

A. Yes, very much so. Ginseng is a wonderful remedy to make you feel full of energy even if you did not sleep, if you are jet lagged, or if you suffer from short-term tiredness for any reason. It will not make you feel hyperactive, jittery, or "wired" as you might feel with stimulants. It will simply help you to function normally and forget that you lack sleep. But again, if the problem is long-term insomnia, ginseng is not the final answer, and you need to deal with the cause of the problem.

Q. Will ginseng help me even if I am not tired?

A. Ginseng is a health remedy that can help the body to run more smoothly. As the Chinese say, it creates a more efficient inner balance. Therefore it can help you even if you are not tired. It can be used as part of a health-maintenance program along with other herbs and self-care measures. The general rule is, the more tired and run-down you feel, the more likely you will notice the effects of ginseng. But if you are not tired and run down, it may still help you, even though you do not notice it. For example, it can aid your immune system, but you may not notice any dramatic changes. How to use ginseng to aid general health is discussed below.

Q. Is there scientific evidence that ginseng can improve energy and wakefulness?

A. Yes, there is. Scientists have studied the effects

of ginseng on animals as well as on human beings.

Research began in Russia, in the late 1940s. Professor Brekhman of the Institute of Biologically Active Sciences in Vladivostok, discovered that many of the health-giving herbs used in traditional Oriental medicine could be tested in the laboratory. Like an engineer who checks the strength of a bridge by testing it under extreme stress, Professor Brekhman decided to test the effectiveness of ginseng in situations of stress. He gave ginseng to mice and measured how long the mice were able to endure a rigorous program of forced exercise. He discovered that mice who were fed ginseng could swim or run for much longer than mice who had not taken ginseng. Even more significant, the mice who took ginseng over a long period of time had even greater physical stamina than those who took it only for a short time. In fact, the longer they took ginseng, the better the result, and it lasted for a while even after ginseng was stopped. This kind of study has been repeated all over the world.

Ginseng improves mental acuity as well as physical stamina. Numerous studies, especially those by Professor Takagi and Dr. Shoji at the University of Tokyo, have shown that animals learn faster and remember better when given ginseng. In experiments, rodents who were fed ginseng showed noticeable improvement in mental stamina. They seemed more active and more inclined to explore their environment. Interestingly, the studies show that laboratory animals given caffeine or other stimulants also move faster and sometimes appear to learn simple tasks more quickly. But when faced with more complex problems, they do better with ginseng and worse with stimulants.

Q. Have scientists studies human beings as well as animals?

A. The effectiveness of ginseng has been researched and verified through scientific studies of human beings, not only animals. The first experiments were tried on soldiers in the Russian army who were asked to participate in a two-mile race. Some took ginseng, while others took a similar-tasting placebo. None of the participants knew which substance they were taking. Those who took ginseng completed the two-mile race in 6 percent less time than their counterparts who had been given the placebo.

This kind of study has been repeated many times. For example, in a study of 100 students at the University of Uppsala, Sweden, ginseng improved test scores on puzzles, brain teasers, and mind-body tests. At the Gentofte University Hospital in Denmark, 112 healthy adults took ginseng for nine weeks. Researchers found that the participants had faster reactions, and they could solve problems more easily than before, although there was no difference in memory and concentration. Studies like these have been extremely convincing. The German government, for example, has acknowledged that ginseng has been proven effective through rigorous scientific study and has licensed ginseng as a medicine to "increase vigor and strength in times of fatigue and debility or declining capacity for work and concentration."

I myself carried out a study at King's College Hospital, London. I tested nurses who were undergoing changes of schedule. They were switching from the day shift to the night shift. I felt that they were excellent candidates for this study, because they were bound to experience some fatigue and stress as their bodies adjusted to a new sleeping schedule. I divided the nurses into two groups. I administered ginseng to the first group and a placebo to the second. On the third day after the switch, both groups were asked to rate their performance, competence, alertness, concentration, and energy level. Virtually all of the ginseng-takers reported improvements in their capacity to cope with their work. The nurses taking the placebo did not report any similar improvement. Interestingly, the nurses taking ginseng slept slightly less than the others, but nevertheless felt better.

Q. If ginseng isn't a stimulant like coffee, then will it still be useful in helping me stay awake after a sleepless night?

A. It certainly will. An early account of ginseng's success was given by Father Jartoux, a French priest who first brought ginseng to the notice of the Royal Society of London in 1714. He wrote that while he was surveying the Chinese border with Korea, a local Mandarin gave him some ginseng. "In an Hour after I found my Pulse much fuller and quicker, I had an Appetite, and found myself much more vigorous and could bear Labour much better and easier than before," he wrote. Later, he rode with the Chinese emperor until he was so exhausted that he could hardly keep himself from falling off his horse. The emperor gave him half a root of ginseng, which he chewed, whereupon he became alert once more and was able to carry on with his activities.

Q. Can ginseng help to boost energy in life-and-death situations and other emergencies?

A. It certainly can. Ginseng has both mental and

physical applications in emergency situations. Chinese soldiers traditionally took ginseng with them into battle. Ginseng helped them to remain alert, focused, and increased their endurance. If they were wounded, ginseng helped them keep going until they could be treated. In the last Vietnamese war, the North Vietnamese used it extensively as an emergency remedy, for example, in cases of shock, loss of blood, and injury. In modern Chinese hospitals, ginseng is used if a patient's blood pressure falls drastically as might happen, for example, after a heart attack. Ginseng will raise the blood pressure and keep the patient going, while the body begins its damage control and repair processes. Ginseng and Eleuthero are used by the Russians and the Chinese to assist people working in difficult and dangerous circumstances, such as deep sea divers, explorers, and commandos in the army.

The use of ginseng as an emergency remedy has a long tradition in Chinese medicine. It is used by those who are so weakened by disease that their life is at risk. Good-quality ginseng can sometimes save lives by boosting vitality, bringing disordered metabolism back into line, and giving the patient a chance to "turn the corner." For people at death's door, the tradition tells us, ginseng can be taken "to keep them going long enough to say goodbye and to sort out their affairs." It would be the one reme-

dy that I would take with me while visiting some-
one very weak, seriously ill, or elderly and ailing. I
have given it to people in intensive care as a liquid
extract and have seen them visibly perk up a couple
of hours later.

3.

How to Boost Performance

In the last chapter, we looked at ginseng as an energy-booster during times of physical or emotional stress. In this chapter, we will look at the well-known use of ginseng and similar herbs in sports, in training, in sexual performance, and in life activities. You will learn about long-term uses of ginseng to enhance performance in an array of different activities in your life.

Q. Can ginseng improve my general performance at work and leisure?

A. Yes. We have seen in the last chapter that ginseng increases wakefulness and energy, and how it helped students, nurses, and others to work more competently at times of high stress and physical demands. Ginseng can also help you build your stamina and heighten your ability to function on a long-term basis.

Q. What's the difference between short-term and long-term use of ginseng?

A. If you need ginseng to help you through an immediate crisis, you should take it only on the morning of the day that you need it. The effect will last for the day. It can help you overcome tiredness and perform at your best, just as it helped Father Jartoux whom we met in the last chapter. So if you have a long day ahead, if you have some challenging assignment, if you have examinations or tests, or if you are faced with a crisis at work, ginseng can be a great help.

For long-term use, you should take ginseng daily for at least a month. The purpose here is to increase your capacity to cope. Ginseng will help you build energy and resistance to the stresses and strains of your demanding work and life. You can take a course of ginseng whenever you go through a difficult period. For example, after a series of experiments at their cosmodrome, Soviet experts in space medicine concluded that ginseng was a better stimulant or tonic for their cosmonauts than the amphetamines used by American astronauts. It increased alertness and performance more successfully, without interfering with normal sleep and without producing hangovers. Soviet cosmonauts took ginseng and eleuthero with them on space missions in the 1970s. These cosmonauts were fit, motivated, energetic young men who took ginseng over a period of time not as a stimulant, but to help them cope with a demanding environment.

Q. Can ginseng increase sports performance?

A. Yes. Ginseng and eleuthero are useful in sports and have been used by many top athletes such as Sebastian Coe, who holds a world record in swimming. Ginseng is used extensively by Olympic athletes, especially those who come from Oriental countries. Soviet athletes and those from Eastern Europe usually use eleuthero. According to the international committee that regulates the use of drugs in sports competitions, use of these herbs is permissible because they are regarded as health tonics rather than performance-enhancing drugs.

Q. What is the most effective use of ginseng in sports training?

A. The most effective use of ginseng is to assist those who are not yet fit to increase their stamina and endurance and to adapt to the rigorous demands of sports training. Ginseng will also be helpful with post-exercise recovery.

Ginseng can also help athletes who are fit and whose bodies are well-toned and energetic. The positive effects of ginseng might not be readily noticeable on the day of a race if the person takes ginseng that morning. However, because it increases vitality, reduces exhaustion, and helps the body adapt to demanding situations, it can help when an athlete is tired, feels below par, or is undergoing particularly intensive training. In these cases, ginseng should be taken for a period of time, such as two months, rather than only on the day of the competition itself.

This is the way ginseng is used in Soviet sports. After a long series of trials at the Lesgraft Institute of Physical Culture and Sports, the director, Professor Anton Korobov, concluded that the action of ginseng-like plants should be "aimed at accelerating the restorative processes after intensive activity and increasing the body's resistance to unfavorable external influence." The result was that Soviet sportsmen were officially instructed by the sports ministry to take ginseng or eleuthero to help overcome exhaustion and stress during training. They continue to take them during sports events, including the Olympics.

Q. What does scientific research say about ginseng and sports?

A. The research generally confirms that the effects of ginseng are most dramatic in people who are building their endurance and stamina, and less noticeable in healthy, energetic young athletes. Sports research was conducted by Professor Forgo at the Cantonal Hospital in Basle, Switzerland. He gave ginseng to groups of athletes and measured their performance on exercise-testing apparatus. Professor Forgo concentrated on such indicators as cardiac output, volume of air in the lungs, amount of oxygen taken in, muscle fatigue, and the efficiency of energy metabolism. Athletes given ginseng showed great improvement in almost all of these signs of fitness, especially the extra oxygen in the lungs and blood. The athletes in these studies took ginseng over a period of nine weeks, and the improvements could be seen for a month or so after they stopped taking ginseng.

Later studies carried out by Dr. Engels and colleagues at Wayne State University Exercise Science Laboratory, Detroit, seemed to contradict these results. Dr. Engels found that healthy young female athletes who took ginseng over a period of two months did not seem to show similar improvement in tests of fitness, exercise capacity, and recovery. A study of fit young marathon runners was carried out at the United States Army Research Institute of Environmental Medicine in Natick, Massachusetts. Some runners took ginseng for one month, while others were given a placebo. At the end of the period, those taking ginseng showed no improvement in stamina and signs of fitness.

It is clear that scientific research presents an unclear and equivocal picture of the effectiveness of ginseng in sports training. Some studies appear to substantiate the claim that ginseng improves stamina in athletes, while other studies appear to contradict that claim. One way of understanding this contradiction in scientific findings is that ginseng has a noticeable effect on people who are not yet physically fit due to age, illness, or stage of athletic training. Athletes who are already physically fit, toned, and energetic do not seem to be affected by ginseng.

Animals studies support these findings. I myself participated in conducting a study at the University of Philadelphia. My colleagues and I found that ginseng definitely helped racehorses to train and increase fitness and endurance. Racehorses who were given ginseng showed greater stamina during practice than racehorses who were not given ginseng. However the ginseng did not necessarily guarantee better performance during the races themselves, once the horses were already fit, toned, and ready for the race.

Q. Is there a difference between ginseng, American ginseng, and eleuthero in improving sports performance?

A. Asian ginseng is best if you are going through difficult, stressful, and demanding times. If you are in a state of real exhaustion and tiredness and must embark upon a course of strenuous athletic training, Asian ginseng will be most helpful.

Eleuthero and American ginseng are gentler. They do not provide as much stimulation or alertness. Instead, they help the metabolism and bodily functions more steadily and invisibly. The end result of increasing vitality and performance may be the same, but eleuthero or American ginseng would be a better choice if you are an athlete already in top shape, who would simply like to give yourself an extra edge over the competition. Eleuthero and

American ginseng, taken over a time, will be as helpful as Asian ginseng in building resistance to stress.

The kind of ginseng you choose might also depend upon your physical and emotional nature. The Chinese tradition differentiates between two different types of people. Asian ginseng is good for people who are, by nature, slower. If you need a great deal of sleep, if you are somewhat on the heavy side, if you tend to get cold easily, if you are more passive than aggressive, if your digestion is sluggish, and if your metabolism is slow, then Asian ginseng is the best choice for you. Your age is also a determining factor: the older you are, the more likely that Asian ginseng will be a more appropriate choice than eleuthero or American ginseng.

Asian ginseng is less appropriate for those who are highly energetic or even nervous, hot blooded, fast in action and thought, need less sleep, and have a fast metabolism and digestion. Young children or even young adults and certainly people of all ages who are hyperactive should take eleuthero or American ginseng if they wish to increase their athletic or general performance. In addition, Asian ginseng tends to be more appropriate for men, while eleuthero and American ginseng work equally well for men and women. In cases of burn-out and complete exhaustion, or in the case of older ages, Asian ginseng is better, whatever your body type or gender.

Q. Is ginseng an aphrodisiac?

A. The short answer is no. Ginseng is certainly found in sex shops and occasionally is joked about. This has led most of the public to view ginseng as "some kind of aphrodisiac." However, the Chinese do not claim that it is a specific sexual stimulant. Instead they use ginseng to maintain potency and virility, which is seen in Eastern culture as a sign of overall good health. Ginseng is used widely in the Orient to combat impotence, especially the decline in virility which occurs with age. Many are impressed by the virility of elderly Chinese people, and the Chinese themselves readily admit that the use of ginseng is partly responsible. So you could take ginseng to combat loss of virility and potency, but not as an aphrodisiac.

The scientific evidence supports this use of ginseng. Animal studies have shown that ginseng can stimulate the production of those sex hormones that ensure normal sexual function and fertility. It does not seem to increase sexual desire in animals or in human beings.

Q. Are there other ways that ginseng can improve function?

A. Yes. Ginseng may improve memory and mental function, but it cannot be called a memory drug. Because it increases alertness, focus, and energy, people who take it might experience greater capacity to absorb and retain information.

4.

Ginseng and Stress

In this chapter, we will explain what stress is, how you can recognize it, and what impact stress has upon your mental and physical health. Then you'll learn how ginseng can help you to cope with the negative effects of stress on your body, and how it can help support your immune system. Lastly, you will learn how to incorporate ginseng and similar herbs into an overall wellness program designed to improve your general health.

Q. What is stress?

A. Stress can be defined as mental or physical tension or strain. The body undergoes stress when it is subjected to extreme physical or emotional exertion, or when it perceives itself to be threatened in some way. Whether the stress is physical or emotional, the body responds in much the same way: the heart speeds up, blood vessels contract, blood pressure rises, metabolism changes, sugar and cholesterol levels rise, the mind becomes exceptionally alert, and muscles become tense.

These responses are excellent for preparing the body for ordinary or even extraordinary physical exertion. If you are a marathon runner, for example, your heart must be toned and able to work more efficiently so as to pump blood. You must be alert and focused. You must be able to metabolize sugar so as to produce the energy necessary to fuel your physical activities. These physical changes are the body's healthy responses to the demands of your exercise regimen.

These responses are also the body's way of preparing you to deal with physical danger. Scientists call these physical reactions the "fight or flight response." If you are about to be attacked by a mad tiger or a crazed gunman, for example, your body will provide you with the energy necessary to fight the menacing force, or to flee it. Your body is being given the means to protect itself from danger.

Unfortunately, in our civilized Western world, the fight or flight response is put into action even when no physical threat is present. The body has automatic responses to any kind of threat, whether it's a real physical attack or a few harsh words at home or in the office. If you get into a fight with your spouse, or if your boss fires you from your job, your body will respond as if the tiger or gunman is about to attack. These responses are coordinated by the nervous system which sets off alarms and high-speed mobilization of the body's defenses. Once the nervous system has alerted the body to danger, the endocrine system becomes involved and hormones are secreted into the body. Hormones are chemical messengers, and the ones involved in the stress response are made in the adrenal glands. During stress, blood is shifted away from "peacetime" functions such as digestion, and the body is mobilized for intense physical activity.

For most of us, the physical activity for which the body is primed is simply not forthcoming. If our employers, colleagues, or family members are angry at us, we cannot physically assault them, nor are we going to run away from them. So the body's defense systems are not properly used, and the person is often unable to relax and allow the systems to return to a healthy state of balance. It is very hard to switch off the intense set of reactions that have been activated. For many people, the state of stress is unremitting and can come from all kinds of directions such as pressure from bosses and deadlines, tension and conflict at home, a nervous or anxious disposition, noisy and distracting work environment, or financial troubles.

Q. What's wrong with stress?

A. Occasional stress is normal, even among people who live a bucolic and quiet lifestyle. Continuous stress, however, is bad for our long-term health. It lowers resistance and immunity, increases blood pressure, and is a cause of digestive disturbances, heart and circulatory problems, cancer, exhaustion, burn-out, insomnia, migraines, headaches, and other disorders. It reduces our general vitality and well-being.

Q. How do I know if I am under stress?

A. Ask yourself some basic questions regarding your life circumstances and your lifestyle. Have you recently undergone any painful experiences, such as loss of a loved one, loss of a job, or marital conflict or friction in some other fundamental relationship? Do you feel your family or work situation to be difficult and filled with pressure and struggle? Do you allow yourself some time for relaxation every day? Is your lifestyle filled with deadlines and pressure?

There are also physical indicators of stress. High blood pressure or blood cholesterol, ulcers and other stomach problems, migraines, insomnia, or chronic fatigue are physical signs of stress. If you are experiencing one or more of these symptoms, you might begin to explore the question of stress in your life.

Q. Can ginseng and similar herbs help me to cope with stress?

A. Herbs such as ginseng can help your body resist stress. They will not, however, change the situation that creates the stress for you. If stress is the symptom of some broader life circumstance, such as a troubled marriage, high-pressure job, or excessively hectic and demanding lifestyle, then the stress should be addressed primarily through examining changes that you can make in your lifestyle. If it is difficult for you to approach the situation on your own, you might consider consulting a trained therapist or counselor to assist you in understanding how you can create a more relaxed lifestyle. However, if stress exists, ginseng and similar herbs can to some extent protect the body from its negative effects.

Q. How do ginseng and similar herbs help the body to deal with stress?

A. Ginseng and similar herbs help the body to adapt to circumstances. This is why they have been described in recent scientific literature as *adaptogens*. An adaptogen is a medicine or herb which assists the body to adapt to an array of different situations. Ginseng and eleuthero have been described as adaptogens because they bring inner balance and harmony to the body. They help you to adapt to change and stress.

Q. What research has been done on adaptogens?

A. The concept of an adaptogen arose through early Russian research on how herbs like ginseng increase resistance to stress in animals, regardless of the nature and source of that stress. Scientists tested stresses such as high or low temperature, radiation, physical exhaustion after extended exercise, toxic drugs and alcohol, loud noises, and metabolic stresses (such as consumption of excess sugar). In all cases, ginseng helped the body to cope much better. Some animals did die, when the stress level exceeded their ability to cope. However, animals given ginseng and similar remedies almost always survived. The scientists found that their glands had more capacity to keep pumping out hormones, and also that the level of hormones in the body was conserved, allowing the animals to keep going for much longer. These findings, which have been replicated in studies with human beings, led to the concept of the adaptogen—an herb that helps to restore and normalize bodily processes.

Soviet cosmonauts took ginseng every day, not only to support their energy, but also to help their body to adapt to a difficult environment. When a Soviet cosmonaut, Alexander Volvov, visited the West after staying in space for 178 days, he told journalists, "We came to share our experience of using this rich and natural medicine. In space it helps us to adapt to weightlessness very quickly and also aids our rehabilitation."

Q. How can an adaptogen like ginseng help me?

A. Because ginseng assists your body in taking in more oxygen, pumping more blood, metabolizing more sugar, and generating more energy, it is helpful in situations that demand a great deal of physical output, such as sports competitions. Ginseng is also helpful when you are under emotional stress, and your body is reacting as if you were being forced to take instantaneous physical action. In such circumstances, your adrenal glands are pouring adrenaline into your system. The adrenaline creates a state of alertness and mobilization of the body's defenses. From a hormonal point of view, you're fighting for your life. If you take ginseng, your adrenal glands secrete less adrenaline and are also able to switch off more easily when the crisis is over. Your body returns to normal more quickly and retains more of its peacetime balance. Consequently less damage is done to your health.

It may come as a surprise to you to realize that tiredness and exhaustion are also stresses. When you push yourself physically, when you exercise beyond the point of exhaustion, or when you deprive yourself of sleep for long periods of time, you create the same set of physical changes as when you are stressed for other reasons. Your body is crying out for sleep and relaxation, but you are driving it to perform and forcing it to ignore the need for rest. The adrenal glands perceive this to be a crisis and react accordingly, pouring adrenaline into the bloodstream. This is responsible for the "second wind" that many people report when they stay up late at night and their tiredness has suddenly disappeared. So the ability of ginseng to restore energy and vitality may be just part of a more general effect on our capacity to handle stress.

Q. What are some of the main research findings on ginseng and stress?

A. A great deal of research has been conducted all over the world. Much of it has concentrated on the changes that happen in the body when ginseng is taken. One of the most interesting studies was carried out in Korea. It demonstrated that under ordinary circumstances, the level of adrenaline and other stress hormones in the blood is generally low. When a stressful situation is encountered, the adrenal glands immediately pump out stress hormones. Then when the stressful crisis is resolved, the hormonal levels slowly return to normal. The same general pattern occurs when ginseng is taken, with one important difference: the stress hormones are not only produced more quickly, but they also disappear from the body more quickly. This is good news, because it is the presence of these hormones in the body well after the physical need for them has expired that causes the damage found in people who have been exposed to long-term stress.

In a study that I conducted at London University, I found that when mice are given ginseng under normal circumstances, their behavior is relatively unchanged. However as soon as they experience stress, such as an exposure to strong light and sound, their reactions and responses become much more intense if they have been given ginseng.

Q. What kinds of stress will respond to ginseng?

A. Ginseng can be helpful in all kinds of stressful situations, as mentioned above. These include times of heavy work, pressure, lack of sleep, sports competitions, and final exams. It can help you through difficult emotional periods in your life. Ginseng also has some additional uses. It has been shown that ginseng can be helpful to people whose bodies have been stressed by substance abuse. There are many studies demonstrating that animals given ginseng or eleuthero cope better with all kinds of poisons and drugs, experiencing fewer negative reactions and side effects. For example, one study showed that ginseng reduced the addictiveness of morphine and helped the liver to dispose of it quickly and safely. There were fewer side effects, but the pain-killing effect of morphine was unchanged. The same holds true for alcohol. If ginseng or eleuthero is taken together with alcohol, the body disposes of the alcohol more quickly, and there are fewer headaches, hangovers, or liver problems. Interestingly, after such studies, Russia started to make a vodka with added eleuthero, and a beer containing eleuthero, which was named "Bodrost" (translating to "good health").

Another stressor to the body is surgery. Indeed, surgery is one of the most stressful experiences the body can undergo. Sometimes, the actual stress itself can create slow recovery and create additional health problems. For example, it is known that the stress of cancer surgery is one of the factors that causes the spread of cancer to other parts of the body, with potentially disastrous consequences for the patient. Studies in Seoul, Korea, with a large number of female patients who had gynecological surgery, showed that if they were given ginseng, their recovery was much faster. All the measures of recovery, such as the proper working of the liver, the production of blood cells, the housecleaning functions of the body, and the immune system, were all restored much faster. Similarly, Russian studies showed that giving eleuthero to children before and after surgery helped to rapidly restore body functions such as body temperature, sugar levels, immune cells, and hormone systems. The children had fewer complications than those who did not get the eleuthero.

Q. Will ginseng help my high blood pressure and elevated blood sugar?

A. Studies have shown that ginseng can moderate the highs and lows of blood sugar levels as well as blood pressure. Ginseng and eleuthero are not the most important or useful remedies against elevated blood pressure or blood sugar problems and fluctuations; however, they are useful additional remedies. They are especially effective if your high blood pressure or high blood sugar is caused by a stressful lifestyle. In a study at the Volga automobile factory in Russia, hundreds of overworked drivers were given eleuthero daily with their tea. The number of drivers with high blood pressure dropped to one-third, compared to what it was before, and compared to drivers who did not take the eleuthero.

So taking an adaptogen like ginseng is an ideal way to protect yourself from high blood pressure and blood sugar caused by stress. These adaptogens should be taken along with other specific treatments and incorporated into a generally healthful lifestyle.

Q. Will ginseng or eleuthero interfere with my current blood pressure medication?

A. Adaptogens do not conflict with conventional drugs or other herbal treatments. In fact, they can add to their effectiveness.

Q. Can ginseng aid the immune system?

A. Yes. Ginseng and eleuthero are both mild immune tonics. They are especially useful when the immune system as a whole is compromised because of stress and long term-exhaustion. There are a large number of studies that have been carried out in Russia and other places showing that eleuthero can help protect the immune system of people whose immunity is damaged by radiation or by chemotherapy for cancer. For example, many studies conducted by Dr. Valery Kupin at Moscow's All-Union Cancer Research Center showed that eleuthero could completely prevent the decline in the white blood cells of the immune system after radiation and chemotherapy. Breast cancer patients survived longer when given eleuthero with their treatment. In every case, the use of eleuthero to support the vital functions of the patients allowed a much higher dose of the drugs to be given, which itself helped the patients to live longer. This has been confirmed by Dr. Phillip Medon at the Northeast Louisiana State University at Monrothat. The studies he conducted demonstrated that eleuthero could aid anticancer drugs in their action on cancer cells by protecting the cells and allowing higher doses to be administered with fewer negative side effects.

I conducted a study with Dr. Ben-Hur at the Israel Nuclear Research Center. We showed that eleuthero could help human cells to recover more quickly and completely from radiation. They were better able to repair the damage to their genetic information. Scientists at INSERM, the French National Research Center, in Villejuif, France, also showed that mice given eleuthero after radiation were much more likely to survive. The cells which made up their blood and immune system were also much more protected. Eleuthero was used extensively after the Chernobyl nuclear accident, to help restore the immune system of those damaged by the radiation.

In one German study, the authors found a "drastic increase in the number of immunocompetent cells" in those volunteers who took Eleuthero for four weeks. The readiness and capacity of the entire immune system were noticeably increased. A study run by Dr. Scaglione of the Department of Pharmacology of the University of Milan in Italy showed an identical pattern was in normal people given ginseng for eight weeks. It is clear that both ginseng and eleuthero are effective at supporting the immune system.

There have been huge Russian studies on the way eleuthero can improve general resistance. In the winter of 1975, more than 13,000 car workers at the Volga car plant were given 2 g per day of eleuthero. The incidence of missed work days due to illness fell by around 40 percent, as compared to workers who did not take eleuthero. In a follow-up seven-year study with truck drivers, 2 g of eleuthero daily significantly decreased the incidence of influenza and influenza symptoms, reducing the number of lost work days.

It is interesting that there is a close connection between feeling good and being resistant to disease. A general attitude of positivity, motivation, and cheerfulness is one of the best tonics for the immune system. We can see that ginseng, which can increase general energy, can therefore help the immunity at the same time.

Q. So how do I take ginseng so as to improve my general health and immunity?

A. According to Oriental tradition, the best way to use ginseng is to embark upon a two-month wellness program. You would be well-advised to regard this time as a period of complete renewal of energy and health. In the Oriental tradition, it is specifically described how to do this—the time when you take a ginseng health course should be the time when you gather and store energy, not expend it. Therefore it should be a time when you consume less food, take regular aerobic exercise, allow yourself a great deal of rest and relaxation, avoid stress as much as possible, do not indulge in alcohol and drugs, and reduce sexual activity. The plan is for you to build your energy reserves. Of course, you can take ginseng to help you cope with crisis situations or to help you alleviate the negative effects of stress and tiredness; but this way, you are not building your energy bank account. You are spending what you put in. For health purposes, you must make minimal withdrawals from the energy bank while ginseng makes maximum deposits. Let ginseng fill up the account. Let ginseng store up energy and vitality that will stay with you for life.

5.

Young Body,
Young Mind

In the West, people look to old age with dread. In the Orient, however, people venerate the elderly and look to old age as a time of fulfillment, wisdom, and strength. In fact, the Chinese define health as arriving at old age vital, active, and virile. They credit ginseng with enabling the elderly population to remain healthy and vigorous. As modern science finds new ways to prolong life, the number of senior citizens in the West is increasing dramatically. For this reason, it is particularly important to find ways that will build health and strength among elderly people. This chapter will address some basic questions about aging. You will learn how you can use ginseng in your youth so as to ensure a healthier old age and a longer life. You will also learn how you can use ginseng if you are already a senior citizen, so as to increase your vitality and prolong your life.

Q. What is aging?

A. Aging is a gradual process of reduced function of all body functions. The organs still work well even in an old person, providing he is healthy. But what declines is the way they all work together. The body's capacity to adapt and adjust declines with age. Things don't work with the same sharpness and tight organization, just as a tape cassette will become fuzzy after many runs through a tape recorder. And there is less energy available to cope with change or threat. For example, the immune system cannot respond so well to bacteria, which is why elderly people tend to be more prone to infectious diseases. The regulation of sugar levels becomes less efficient, so many older people begin to suffer from mild diabetes.

Aging is not a disease. It is a natural process. While it cannot be stopped, it can be slowed, and we have the ability to live a long, healthy life until our natural lifespan has run its course. An old person need not have diseases of the heart and circulation, of memory, or of the joints. Our target should be to arrive at old age running, not crawling. If our bodies could be strengthened, we could live to our maximum lifespan without being ravaged by age-associated diseases. And this maximum would be much more than the average lifespan of seventy-five years. For example, there are areas of the world where people live a long and healthy life, with very few diseases, and it is common in these communities to find people well over a hundred years old.

Q. What are some of the ways in which I can reach a healthy old age?

A. In general, any treatment that improves health and fitness can be expected to aid in resisting the effects of aging. Yoga and exercise can increase life span and improve the chances of a fit, disease-free, and vital old age. It is also important to keep the body free of toxins. That means avoiding junk food; reducing consumption of animal products and animal fat; avoiding processed foods, instant meals, food containing additives and preservatives; and reducing intake of caffeine, sugar and soft drinks. The diet should be based on fresh vegetables, fruit, whole grains, legumes, soy products, and other wholesome and nutritious foods.

The communities of people who live extraordinarily long and healthy lives tend to have much in common, no matter what part of the world they are located. They eat a frugal diet of wholesome food, grown without chemical pesticides. They do not

have any processed foods. They are generally agri-
cultural workers who engage in physical labor all
their lives. They live in the clean air of hilly regions
in which they walk everywhere without cars. They
live a stress-free life in accordance with natural
rhythms. They use natural plant remedies to maintain health when needed. Westerners would be well
advised to incorporate as many components of this
natural lifestyle into their own lives, so as to ensure
maximum health and vigor during old age.

Q. Is ginseng regarded as a remedy to prolong life?

A. Very much so. It may be one of the most important that we know. The Chinese, of course, have a rich
source of various herbal medicines that are useful in
combating the symptoms of aging, but none has the
same reputation as ginseng. In China, Mao Zedong
and Chou en-Lai were both known to take ginseng
regularly, and they lived a remarkably long life. In
1933, *The New York Times* carried a story about a
Peking professor who lived for 256 years. It is of interest that he attributed his purported longevity to the
ginseng tea he brewed daily. The herbal manuals are
insistent that ginseng can prolong life, although they
recognize that it certainly is not the fabled Elixir of
Immortality.

Q. How can ginseng help me to reduce the signs of aging?

A. Both in Chinese medicine and the modern view, aging is a process of increasing inner disorganization and inefficiency. Any agent or activity that improves the body's harmony and tunes the body's engines ought to slow aging. This is the way ginseng works. It reduces stress, improves efficiency, and helps the hormones to regulate bodily functions. So there is less inner wear and tear as we age.

Ginseng can slow the aging process; and, perhaps more importantly, it can dramatically effect the way we age. Most people experience more and more episodes of poor health as they get older. They seem to suffer from increased fatigue and to have less energy. Both of these symptoms of aging can be helped by ginseng. It is my belief that the Chinese have introduced to the world the only remedy ever shown to have medicinal powers that specifically fit the conditions of the elderly.

Q. Is there any scientific evidence for ginseng as an anti-aging remedy?

A. There is certainly evidence that points to ginseng as an anti-aging remedy; however, that evidence is not conclusive as yet. It would be difficult to demonstrate the effect of a medication on the life span of human beings, because doing so would take so long that the scientists might not be alive at the end of the experiment. At the University of London, my colleagues and I have tried to check if ginseng helps animals to live longer. Mice were given very small doses of ginseng throughout life. The treated mice appeared more active than those not given ginseng, however we could not detect any increase in lifespan. A similar study conducted in Russia produced more positive results. Soviet scientists reported that a colony of rats given higher doses of ginseng lived considerably longer than a similar colony without ginseng. More research needs to be conducted for scientifically valid conclusions to be reached.

A more productive and conclusive avenue of research has been on human cells that have been removed from the body. In experiments, I have shown (as have other scientists) that ginseng can delay the aging of cells and improve their survival under stress.

There have been some suggestive and encouraging studies performed on older people. Trials of ginseng among the elderly in hospitals and old-age homes have yielded encouraging results. In one case, sixty-six patients were given ginseng and vitamins. Improvements were noticed in most of those who suffered from cardiovascular diseases, depression, and reduced vitality. Many of the patients showed an awakening interest in life. Such psychological benefits are also the most marked feature of a German clinical trial of ginseng among ninety-five patients in old-age homes. Besides improvements in blood pressure, memory, neurological function, and bodily function, fifty-eight of the patients showed "an enhancement of mood so marked as to be almost euphoric, and in almost all cases it was maintained for a period of months." The doctors continue: "It goes without saying that tiredness or exhaustion were among our patients' main symptoms. . . . 83 percent showed clear improvements in both these syndromes, which can be considered an excellent result."

I set up a study at St. Francis Hospital in London on sixty senior citizens who complained of being tired and run down. For ten days they took ginseng. I waited a few weeks, then gave them a placebo for another ten days. Neither the participants nor the nurse who evaluated them knew which course of treatment involved authentic ginseng, and which involved the placebo. We found that people who took ginseng had a clear improvement in alertness, speed of reaction, and coordination at tasks that we set for them. Some of them said they felt more energetic and active. They did not experience similar improvement when they took the placebo.

Q. So how do I take ginseng against signs of aging?

A. Begin by obtaining the best ginseng available. Ideally, it should be the whole root, or a paste extract of Oriental red ginseng. (I'll explain more about this in Chapter 7.) To help with aging, you need the stimulating, vitalizing potency of real Asian ginseng, rather than eleuthero or other Oriental tonic herbs. As you move through middle age, begin to take ginseng for a period of one to two months every year, as advised in the previous chapter. As you begin to approach old age, you can take ginseng daily.

Always remember that ginseng is not a panacea nor a magic elixir of immortality. It will not, all by itself, ensure health and vitality. Basic methods of keeping fit and healthy must go along with ginseng. Ginseng cannot be a substitute for wise living.

Q. What can I expect when I take ginseng for aging?

A. Ginseng can reduce the effects of aging in a mild and gentle manner, building up over a long period of time. You should be aware that people will vary considerably in their response to it, depending on such factors as individual constitution, diet, and lifestyle. One person may feel the effects of ginseng immediately, another may not. In one case it may have a profound effect on hormones, in another case on immunity. Each person's reaction will be idiosyncratic and highly particular to the individual, but it's clear that ginseng will exert a powerfully positive impact, no matter what your constitution might be. It can add years to your life and improve the quality of living during those extra years.

6.

Ginseng's Myth,
Legend, and History

There is a rich cultural tradition about ginseng, mostly from China and Korea. But the Native Americans also had their legends about the American cousin. These stories and myths are not just for our entertainment. They can actually be very instructive in helping us understand how to best use ginseng. In this chapter, you will learn what the ancient Oriental herbal experts said about ginseng, and what they used it for. You will meet wild ginseng and understand why the price of a single root of wild ginseng can be as much as $10,000. You will read stories about the discovery of ginseng, how it is hunted and harvested, and what it looks like. You will also learn about the fascinating history of ginseng in America.

Q. How was ginseng discovered?

A. The real story is lost in the mists of time. But the legendary discoverer of ginseng is well known to all Chinese, an essential part of Chinese folk lore. He is called the Emperor Shen Nung, the mythological discoverer of herbal medicine as well as agriculture. He wrote the first book on Chinese herbs, called the *Shen Nung Pen Tshao Tching* (translated as *The Celestial Cultivator's Guide to the Understanding of Remedies*). This book dates back more than 2,000 years. Many of the health-giving remedies in Shen Nung's list are still used today. Ginseng was one of his greatest discoveries. He is supposed to have had an extraordinary skill at discovering remedies. One legend states that he discovered more than fifty new remedies in one day alone through wandering about and meeting the plants, sensing their quality, tasting them, and coming to an understanding of their healing power. It is no accident that he was both a healer and a farmer, because both vocations are based on the art of maintaining health. A good doctor, in the Chinese tradition, is skilled at keeping people healthy. A good farmer is skilled at preventing disease in crops and animals.

There are many legends and stories which portray the discovery of ginseng as something close to a miracle. In one story, the entire village of Shantang in Shensi province was disturbed every night by a strange howling. Unable to stand it, all the villagers gathered one night and followed the sound. They found that the sound emanated from a plant, which they began to dig up. They discovered a huge, man-shaped root that had been calling for attention. The root was named "spirit of the earth."

Eleuthero was always known in Chinese medicine, where it was called *ciwuja*. It was used traditionally there as a mild tonic, but never as well known and widely used as ginseng. It was rediscovered recently in Russia, not by herbalists but by scientists. A young medical doctor named Gorovoy noticed that deer were greedily eating the leaves of a large thorny shrub in the forest. He brought it in for study in the laboratory. Gorovoy found it to have ginseng-like effects, since it increased the stamina of mice.

Q. What do the traditional Oriental herbalists say about ginseng?

A. The most ancient description of the effects of ginseng remains the best description we have to date. Shen Nung wrote that ginseng "tastes sweetish and its property is slightly cooling. It grows in the gorges of the mountains. It is used for repairing the five organ systems, harmonizing energies, strengthening the soul, reducing fear, removing toxic substances, brightening the eyes, opening the heart, and improving thought. Continuous use will invigorate the body and prolong life." This is a remarkably complete and accurate description of ginseng's effects, covering most of the actions of ginseng that we have described in this book, and that have been verified by modern scientific research. The phrase "strengthening the soul and reducing fear" might translate into the modern concept of enabling the person to cope with stress.

A more recent description in one of the herbal guides used in Oriental medicine states that ginseng "nourishes and strengthens the body, stops vomiting, clears thinking, removes weakness, and [heals] other mind-body problems. In a word, it gives a vigorous tone to the body even in old age."

We have to allow for some poetic license in these claims. They extol the virtues of a substance held in reverence, while simultaneously advising people regarding its use. Because ginseng is regarded as almost sacred, descriptions tend to go over the top. There is no plant that is held in so much awe by so many people. It is loved and cherished throughout the Far East. Wars have been fought among the Tartars for possession of ginseng lands. Fabulous prices were paid for wild ginseng in Imperial times: an old root would fetch 250 times its weight in silver.

Q. Can I obtain this amazing and highly valuable ginseng root in my local health food store?

A. No. The incredible appreciation of the Chinese for ginseng is for the root that is grown in the wild and found in the forest. Wild ginseng is virtually extinct today. An occasional wild root is sometimes discovered in the forests of Eastern China. It makes its way to Hong Kong, where fabulous prices are paid for it, even today. Cultivated ginseng is acknowledged to have much weaker properties than the wild root. It is much cheaper and is the only kind that we find on sale locally.

Q. What does Native American tradition have to say about American ginseng?

A. The Native American healers respected ginseng, although American ginseng was never seen with the same degree of reverence as it was in China. The Iroquois regarded it simply as a root which helped the digestive process and metabolism of food. The Menonini and the Cherokees called ginseng "the little man." They used it as a general tonic, as well as for menstrual problems. Several tribes used it for shortness of breath and as an aid for the wounded. Later on, during the early part of the nineteenth century, many of the Indian medicines were incorporated into the herbal books and American official drug lists. Ginseng was described there as a root that aids the stomach and helps with internal injuries. Some of the early herbal botanists did note that American ginseng was not a stimulant like its Asian cousin, although it was a useful mild tonic. Unlike Asian ginseng, the American root has never been gathered to extinction, and it is now a protected species in America. For this reason, it is found wild even today. Large quantities of the wild root, and even more of the cultivated American ginseng, are exported every year to China where they are bought as less stimulating alternatives to Asian ginseng.

It is possible that wild American ginseng is more powerful than cultivated Asian ginseng. Certainly, they are of comparable quality and effectiveness, although American ginseng is a less potent stimulant than Asian cultivated ginseng. Both have harmonizing and immune-supporting effects, which were noticed by the Native Americans as well as the Chinese.

Q. Is it true that Daniel Boone earned his living trading American ginseng?

A. Daniel Boone collected ginseng in the forest. He also bought a great deal more from white settlers. In 1787, he went up the Ohio river in a boat which carried nearly fifteen tons of wild American ginseng. The boat overturned, and he lost it all. Undismayed, he went back and collected an equivalent amount by the next year. He made much money from ginseng, which he sold to traders on the East Coast, who in turn sold it to the Chinese.

Q. What impact did ginseng have on American history?

A. Ginseng led to a great deal of trade between China and America. The American ginseng exports began early that century with reports that American ginseng could be dug up in the forests of Canada and North America. This brought the Chinese to Canada. They started a ginseng rush. From the eighteenth century onwards, American ginseng was intensively collected by Native Americans as well as white settlers. It was overcollected in Canada without any replanting, and so it became rare there.

The trade moved to North America, where villagers and fur trappers all went out with mattock and sack to search for *seng*, as they called it. The seng was bought by the fur traders, and huge profits were made. The amounts were staggering. More than 622,761 pounds of dried wild American ginseng roots were exported in 1862. At the end of the nineteenth century, wild ginseng became harder to find, and cultivation began in forest gardens that mimicked the shaded forest hillsides in which ginseng grew naturally.

7.

Buying and Using Ginseng

This chapter is your comprehensive guide to taking ginseng. You will learn which kinds of ginseng are available and which are preferable, as well as how much to take and how to take it. You will be introduced to the various ginseng products and will find out which brands are most effective, and where you can obtain them.

Q. How is ginseng cultivated and processed?

A. Ginseng is cultivated in beds and under shade nets that imitate the shaded forest. It is grown from seeds that take two years to germinate. The seedlings are planted in deep beds of fertile and well-drained soil, with a straw or leaf mulch.

Ideally, the ginseng roots should be grown in the beds for four to five years before they are dug up. In the traditional methods, the ginseng roots are transplanted by hand almost every year to avoid fungi and other pests that attack the roots. Today, however, unfortunately fungicides and pesticides are used instead. These contain chemicals which can contaminate the roots. To avoid the need for chemical fungicides and pesticides, ginseng growers often harvest the roots while they are still young.

After harvest, the roots are washed, graded, and dried. The dried roots are a light yellow-beige color. Larger, good quality roots from some premium farms are steamed before drying. This gives the roots a red, glassy appearance. These roots are described as red ginseng, while the unsteamed roots are known as white ginseng. The hairs and side-branches of the roots are removed and sold separately as root hairs.

Many companies from all over the world make extracts of the roots. These concentrated extracts are made by grinding the roots and mixing them for some time in a bath of water and alcohol. After this, the extract is concentrated and all its water and alcohol evaporated away to give a powdered extract.

Q. What are the best quality roots?

A. Here are a few guidelines to assist you in shopping for ginseng roots.

- The older the root—that is, the longer it has been growing—the better. Old roots are especially effective at helping the immune system and general health. The best roots available in the market today are five to six years old. They are about five inches long.
- Red ginseng is usually better than white, because only the best quality and oldest roots are used for steaming. Steaming helps to preserve some of the medicinal constituents.
- If you cannot obtain red ginseng roots, you might be able to find good quality Chinese white ginseng. Be aware that Japanese red ginseng if often quite poor in quality.
- The root body is better than the tails, hair, and pieces.
- Probably the best ginseng today comes from Korea, which has government controls and standards in place for the industry. Second best is China, and third best is Japan.
- It is possible to obtain wild American ginseng in the United States. This is better quality than

cultivated American ginseng.
- Good ginseng should taste rich, strong, and bitter, with an undertone of sweetness. If it has no taste, don't buy it.

Q. How should I use the ginseng root?

A. My recommendation is that for long-term regular use you take a dose of approximately 2 g of root daily, split into morning and evening doses. You can double the dose for immediate or short term use, for example, as a stimulant to combat fatigue and exhaustion, in cases of weakness during convalescence, or while going through a period of stress.

Remember that dosage is to some extent an individual matter, depending on factors such as constitution, the reason for taking ginseng, diet, age, and state of health. People should try to find the dose that is right for them by starting low and increasing the dosage until they hit the level at which they notice positive effects. A course of ginseng should last for at least a month. Older people can take ginseng continuously for a long time.

Q. Where can I obtain ginseng roots?

A. If you want top quality ginseng, go to Chinatown or the Chinese shops and buy the best quality red ginseng root that you can afford. If you cannot obtain red ginseng, try to find the oldest white roots you can, according to the guide given in this chapter.

Q. What if I can't obtain ginseng roots?

A. If the ginseng root is unobtainable, then the next best ginseng products are Korean or Chinese imported extracts. These are thick and dark in appearance and are highly concentrated.

If you cannot obtain authentic imported extracts, then you should use powdered extracts or ground root in capsules or tablets. These are the conventional ginseng supplements that you can buy in any health foods store or pharmacy. Most of these products, made by reputable companies, are comparable in effectiveness. I recommend that you choose capsules or tablets described as "standardized," because they guarantee constant potency (by chemical analysis) in every dose. They should report a certain percentage of ginsenosides (the active ingredients) on the label.

The least effective products are the instant ginseng teas, candy, cosmetics, soups, and ginseng soft drinks. These contain very little active ginseng in them. Ginseng cosmetics are not effective. Ginseng needs to be taken internally to work.

Q. How should I take ginseng?

A. The ginseng root is very hard, and it may be necessary to use a hammer to break off a usable piece. There are two ways to use the chunk of ginseng that you have broken off. You can chew a piece of the right size until it is completely dissolved in the mouth. You can also take ginseng in the traditional way, as the Chinese have done for centuries—to boil the ginseng in a small pot for several hours, and then drink the liquid. A ceramic or glass pot is better than metal for the purpose. The Chinese traditionally boil it overnight, then get up early, drink the ginseng tea, and go back to bed. Another traditional approach is to soak some good ginseng root in brandy for a couple of weeks, and take a nip now and then.

Use ginseng products as directed on the packet. However read the packets carefully to distinguish extracts from powdered root. With products containing extracts, take an amount equivalent to 2 to 4 g of actual root. With products containing ground root powder, take 2 to 4 g of the product itself. Often the dosage recommendations on the packets are too low.

Q. How safe is ginseng?

A. Ginseng is remarkably safe, even in large doses or when taken over a long period of time. This has been confirmed by modern research. Professor Brekhman of the Institute of Biologically Active Sciences in Vladivostok, found that animals had to consume a voluminous quantity of ginseng if they were to suffer any negative results. A harmful dose for animals has been shown to be at least 1,000 times more than the recommended dose for human beings. A man would have to consume three to four pounds of pure ginseng at one sitting in order to suffer dangerous effects. Research studies on human patients have never revealed any harmful effects. Monitoring agencies such as the Food and Drug Administration accept that ginseng is safe and allow it to be sold without restriction.

It is nevertheless important to realize that ginseng is a medicine, and there are no medicines that don't have some unwanted effects under some conditions. No medicine should ever be abused. A recent survey conducted by an American doctor showed that some young people who had been taking excessive amounts of ginseng for long periods of time experienced some negative symptoms, including insomnia, over-excitation, nausea, and elevated blood pressure. One reason for these side effects could be that the young people also consumed large quantities of caffeine, thereby becoming overstimulated. The Chinese tradition states that the young and healthy need no more than an occasional course of ginseng, and only the sick, debilitated, and aged may take it all the time. Healthy, energetic, or hyperactive people who take large quantities of ginseng over extended periods of time, especially if they are also using some other kind of stimulant such as caffeine, can experience symptoms of overstimulation.

For best effects, Asian ginseng should be taken in autumn or winter rather than in the heat of summer.

Conclusion

Although ginseng is one of the best of Oriental medicines, it has taken thousands of years to appear in Western pharmacies and stores. The reason for the discrepancy between Eastern and Western use of this extraordinary remedy is that it has been misunderstood by modern Western medicine, which is used to stronger, curative drugs.

Ginseng, like many other herbs, has a more subtle effect than modern medicines or stimulants such as caffeine, but it can help you in ways that are more healthy and long-lasting. It is the best of all tonic medicines, a safe, health-enhancing herb that can aid energy, vitality, performance, and activity. Its most dramatic and profound effects are on those who are neediest—people suffering from exhaustion, stress, burn-out, convalescence, chronic fatigue, or other symptoms associated with aging.

There are gaps in conventional medicine, and one of them is the inability to find safe and effective remedies to help us cope with the stress of modern life and to support our health and vitality. Herbs such as ginseng fill this gap. Herbs should be used as safe, in-home treatments for mild common health problems or as restoratives and tonics to maintain health, while the stronger medicines should be used when a serious illness strikes. In this way, ancient wisdom and modern science will work hand-in-hand toward better health and vigor.

Glossary

Adaptogen. A substance that helps systems in the body to adjust to stress and imbalance.

Adrenal glands. Glands that lie just above the kidneys and are responsible for making and sending out the hormones that organize the body's response to stress.

Aphrodisiac. A substance that specifically increases sexual desire and sexual energy.

Hormones. Chemical substances that circulate through the body and co-ordinate and regulate all aspects of the body's work.

Metabolism. The flow and exchange of bodily chemicals, such as sugars, that create energy and sustain the activities of life.

Stress. Continuous demands on body and mind

that damage health by creating a long-term state of alarm within the body.

Restorative. A remedy that does not cure specific symptoms, but rather restores energy and activity, especially in situations such as convalescence.

Traditional medicine. The ancient systems of medicine that offer many alternative solutions to health problems and are gentler and safer than those offered by conventional medicine.

Vitality. A deep source of energy and well-being that keeps us feeling healthy and vigorous.

References

Chong SKF and Oberholzer VG, "Ginseng—is there a use in clinical medicine?," *Postgraduate Medical Journal* 64 (1988): 841-846.

Hallstrom C, Fulder S, and Carruthers M, "Effect of ginseng on performance of nurses on night Duty," *Comparative Medicine East and West* 6 (1982): 277-282.

Lewis W, "Ginseng: a medical enigma" In: *Plants in Indigenous Medicine & Diet: Biobehavioral Approaches*, ed. Etkin, N.L. (Bedford Hills, NY: Redgrave Publishing,1986).

Liu CX, and Xiao PG, "Recent advances on ginseng research in China," *Journal of Ethnopharmacology* 36 (1992): 27-38.

Ng TB, and Yeun HW, "Scientific basis of the therapeutic effects of ginseng," In *Folk Medicine: The Art and the Science*, ed. Steiner RP (Washington: American Chemical Society, 1986).

Ussher J. et al., "The relationship between health related quality of life and dietary supplementation in British middle managers: a double-blind placebo controlled study," *Psychology and Health* 10 (1995) 97-111.

Bittles AH, Fulder SJ, Grant EC, and Nicholls MR, "The effect of ginseng on the lifespan and stress response in mice," *Gerontology* 25 (1978): 125-131.

Ben-Hur E, and Fulder SJ, "Effect of panax ginseng saponins and eleutherococcus senticosus on survival of cultured mammalian cells after ionizing irradiation," *American Journal of Chinese Medicine* 9 (1981): 48-56.

RJ, "Siberian Ginseng (eleutherococcus senticosus maxim)," *British Journal of Phytotherapy* 2 (1991): 61-71.

Suggested Readings

Fulder S. *The Book of Ginseng and Other Chinese Herbs for Vitality*. Rochester, VT: Healing Arts Press, 1993.

Fulder S. *The Ginseng Book*. Garden City Park, NY: Avery Publishing Group, 1996.

Kaptchuk T. *The Web That Has No Weaver*. New York, NY: St. Martins Press, 1984.

Prevention Magazine. *Prevention's Food and Nutrition*. New York, NY: Berkeley Books, 1990.

Teeguarden R. *Chinese Tonic Herbs*. Tokyo and New York: Japan Publications, 1984.

Yutis P and Walker M. *The Downhill Syndrome*. Garden City Park, NY: Avery Publishing Group, 1997.

Index

Adaptogens, 46–48
Adrenal glands, reaction
  to stress, 48, 49
Aging
  ginseng and, 60–65
  what it is, 58–59
American ginseng
  description of, 13–14
  historical impact of,
    73–74
  historical use of, 71–72
  use in sports, 37–38
  See also Ginseng;
    Eleuthero.
Araliaceae, 12
Asian ginseng. *See*
  Ginseng.

Ben-Hur, E., 54
Blood pressure. *See* High
  blood pressure.
Blood sugar. *See* Elevated
  blood sugar.

Brekhman, Professor, 25,
  81

Caffeine, 11. *See also*
  Coffee.
Celestial Cultivator's Guide
  to the Understanding of
  Remedies (Nung), 68
Ciwuja, 69. *See also*
  Eleuthero.
Coffee, as a stimulant,
  21–22. *See also* Caffeine.
Cultivated ginseng. *See*
  Ginseng.

Eleuthero, 29
  adaptogen, as an, 46
  discovery of, 69
  high blood pressure and,
    52–53
  immune system, effect
    on, 53–55
  sports and use of, 33,

37–38
substance abuse and,
 50–51
surgery and, 51
what it is, 14
See also American ginseng; Ginseng.
Eleutherococcus. See
 Eleuthero.
Elevated blood sugar, 52
En-Lai, Chou, 60
Encyclopedia Britannica, 16
Engels, Dr., 35

Forgo, Professor, 35

Ginseng
 adaptogen, as an, 46,
  47–48
 aging and, 60–65
 aphrodisiac, as an, 39
 blood pressure, effect on,
  29, 52
 caffeine, compared with,
  11, 20, 21–22
 constituents of, 15
 cultivation of, 75–76
 effects of, 16–17
 energy booster, as an,
  19–30(?)
 emergency remedy, as an,
  28–30
 high blood pressure and,

52–53
how to take, 78, 80–81
immune system, effect
 on, 54–55
impotence, for, 39
insomnia and, 23–24
jet lag and, 23
legends of, 68–69, 69–71
long-term use of, 10,
 32–33, 78
main use of, 19–20
memory and, 40
mental function and, 25,
 40
panacea, as a, 15–16
physical effects of, 16–17
plant, 12–13
shopping for, 77–78
short-term use of, 10,
 32–33
side-effects, 81–82
species of, 13–14
sports, use in, 33, 34,
 35–37, 37–38
stimulant, as a, 20, 21,
 32–33
stress and, 11, 45, 46,
 49–51
substance abuse and,
 50–51
supplements, 79–80
surgery and, 51
tonic, as a, 11

where it grows, 13
See also American ginseng; Eleuthro.
Ginseng extract. *See* Ginseng.
Ginseng plant. *See* Ginseng.
Ginseng root. *See* Ginseng.
Ginsenosides, 15

Herbs
  adaptogens, as, 46
  stress and, 45–46
High blood pressure, 52–53
Himalayan ginseng, 14

Immune system, ginseng's effect on, 53–55
Impotence, 39
Insomnia, 23–24

Jet lag, 23

Korobov, Anton, 34
Kupin, Valery, 53

Mendon, Phillip, 54

New York Times, The, 60
Nung, Emperor Shen, 68

Oura, Professor, 21

Panax ginseng, 6, 12. *See also* Ginseng.
Panax quinquefolium, 14. *See also* American ginseng.
Physical effects of ginseng use, 16–17

Red ginseng. See Ginseng.

San ch'i ginseng, 14
Scaglione, Dr., 54
Shen Nung Pen Tshao Tching (Nung), 68
Shogi, Dr., 25
Shori, Deepak, 21
Siberian ginseng. *See* Eleuthero.
Sports and use of ginseng, 33, 34–35, 35–37
Stimulants, 21–22
Stress
  adaptogens for stress, 46
  adrenal glands and, 48, 49
  ginseng for stress, 45, 49–51
  herbs for stress, 45–46
  indicators of stress, 44–45
  physical reactions, 42–43
  results of continuous stress, 44

what it is, 41
Substance abuse, 50–51

Takagi, Professor, 25

*United States National
   Formulary*, 16

White ginseng. *See*

Ginseng.
Wild American ginseng.
   See American ginseng.
Wild ginseng, 71

Zedong, Mao, 60